YOUR KNOWLEDGE HAS VALUE

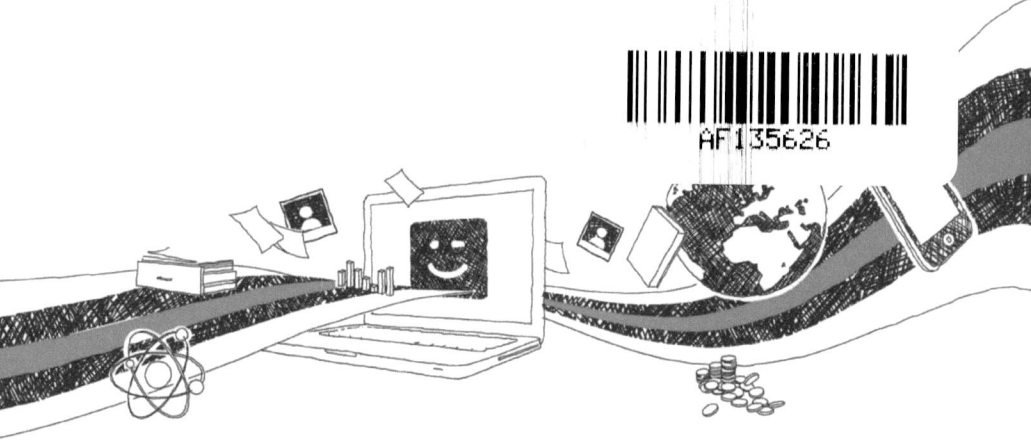

- We will publish your bachelor's and master's thesis, essays and papers

- Your own eBook and book - sold worldwide in all relevant shops

- Earn money with each sale

Upload your text at www.GRIN.com and publish for free

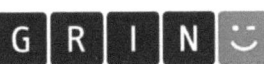

Strategic planning & OHSMS performance measurements and calculations

Damien Hiquet

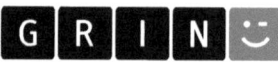

Bibliographic information published by the German National Library:

The German National Library lists this publication in the National Bibliography; detailed bibliographic data are available on the Internet at http://dnb.dnb.de.

ISBN: 9783346682376
This book is also available as an ebook.

© GRIN Publishing GmbH
Nymphenburger Straße 86
80636 München

Print and binding: Books on Demand GmbH, Norderstedt, Germany
Printed on acid-free paper from responsible sources.

The present work has been carefully prepared. Nevertheless, authors and publishers do not incur liability for the correctness of information, notes, links and advice as well as any printing errors.

GRIN web shop: https://www.grin.com/document/1247254

Strategic planning & OHSMS performance measurements and calculations

D. Hiquet

Table of contents

1. Introduction _____3

2. Strategic planning_____3

3. OHSMS performance measurements and calculations _____9

3.1 Lag indicators _____11

3.1.1 Total Recordable Injury (and illness) (TRI)_____11

3.1.2 Days away / restricted / transfer rate (DART) _____11

3.1.3 Lost Time Injury (LTI)_____12

3.2 Leading indicators _____14

4. Conclusion_____15

References _____16

1. Introduction

The purpose of this essay is to analyse how to incorporate the best way possible the Occupational Health and Safety Management System (OHSMS) in the strategic planning of an organisation, to benefit all its stakeholders and to measure its performance through safety key performance indicators (KPIs).

However, the list of KPIs available to an organisation is not limited to the ones selected for this essay.

Moreover, this exercise underlines the difficulty and challenge to use some indicators or measure their performance.

2. Strategic planning

The Balanced Scoreboard Institute (2021) defines strategic planning as:

> An organizational management activity that is used to set priorities, focus energy and resources, strengthen operations, ensure that employees and other stakeholders are working toward common goals, establish agreement around intended outcomes/results, and assess and adjust the organization's direction in response to a changing environment. It is a disciplined effort that produces fundamental decisions and actions that shape and guide what an organization is, who it serves, what it does, and why it does it, with a focus on the future.

Therefore, it does not only describes the aim of an organisation but also sets the organisation for success.

Most people are visual learners implying that a picture of the strategy of the organisation is understood better by all stakeholders than a written narrative.

Through a balanced scorecard (BSC) organisations:
• Communicate what they are trying to accomplish
• Align the day-to-day work that everyone is doing with strategy
• Prioritise projects, products, and services
• Measure and monitor progress towards strategic targets

This holistic framework for managing strategic plans gives organisations a visible connection between the projects that staff are working on.

In 'figure 1', the mapping of the strategy describes logically the cause-and-effect connection between strategic objectives (i.e., oval shapes).

Editor's note: Image has been removed due to copyright reasons.

Figure 1: Strategy map (Visual Paradigm, n.d.)

This approach is not only about measuring performance but also a way for organisations to try to accomplish their mission, vision, and strategy.

Furthermore, the BSC is an ideal place to identify and mitigate overlooked risks that threaten an organisation carrying out its mission ('figure 2').

Risk Type	Description
Strategic	The risks arising from the Group's implementation of business plans, strategies, decision-making, or resource allocation. They may also relate to governance or changes in the business environment.
Operational	The risks on operations resulting from people, processes and systems (internal operating environment) or from the external operating environment. It includes operational safety and people safety risks.
Financial	The risk of financial loss resulting from fuel price, foreign exchange rate or interest rate fluctuations, or those arising from financial management processes such as credit, liquidity and capital or errors in accounting and reporting.
Legal and Compliance	The risks of non-compliance with the domestic or international regulatory or legal obligations. It includes Corporate Social Responsibility obligations.

Figure 2: Risks treating the organisation

There are external and internal drivers for an organisation to implement a framework.

Indeed, the external pressure comes from regulators, rating agencies, stock exchanges, institutional investors, oversight bodies, competition, globalisation and so on implying more transparency in corporate governance and strict compliance with laws and regulations (Dafikpaku, 2011, as cited in Meng & Yahanpath, n.d.).

Meanwhile, the organisation's internal motivations reside in its perception of the risk.

Rather than seeing it as a negative event, organisations must embrace the risk as an opportunity to leverage the benefits of effectively managing the organisations' risks (Meng & Yahanpath, n.d.).

Moreover, developing an Enterprise Risk Management Enterprise (ERM) plan provides visibility into the universe of risks that could impact the mission of the organisation stated in its strategic plan (Deloitte, 2017).

Thus, ERM is defined as:

A discipline that addresses the full spectrum of an organization's risks, including
challenges and opportunities, and integrates them into an enterprise-wide, strategically
aligned portfolio view. ERM contributes to improved decision making and supports the
achievement of an organization's mission, goals, and objectives (Stanton, 2020).

In 'figure 3', the framework is aligned to AS/NZS ISO 31000:2018 Risk Management –
Guidelines.

Editor's note: Image has been removed due to copyright reasons.

Figure 3:AS/NZS ISO 31000:2018 Risk Management – Guidelines.

The purpose of this process is to communicate in a common language and formally
establish a methodology for identifying, assessing and managing risk in a systematic way

but, also the responsibilities for risk management across the organisation with clear accountabilities for governance.

For instance, implementing mechanisms for formal reporting of risk information and a system assuring the Board that key risks are being managed effectively.

However, the discipline is recent and its implementation is complex. Only a few organisations have successfully implemented an ERM that met expectations (Beasley, Branson, & Hancock, 2010; Locklear, 2012, as cited in Meng & Yahanpath, n.d.).

For example, in the case of Pike River Coal (PRC) in 2010, the Royal Commission on the Pike River Coal Mine Tragedy (2012) recognised that PRC had implemented an integrated control-based risk management framework.

Despite the knowledge by the executive team of the risk of wind-blast and large goaf falls and the reporting of excess methane by the miners, PRC neither suspended hydro extraction nor effectively controlled methane.

Therefore, PRC did not manage risks for other stakeholders (i.e., employees) implying that its ERM framework served only the interests of shareholders as stated in its corporate governance disclosure statement filed with the NZX describing the role of ERM as "an essential part of the company's approach to creating long-term shareholder value" (Pike River Coal Limited, 2010, as cited in (Meng & Yahanpath, n.d.).

Still, the combination of ERM and BSC improves the daily organisational performance, governance, stakeholders' satisfaction and company value by aligning all stakeholders with the organisation's vision, mission and cores values (Cooper, n.d.).

In the BSC, objectives are identified for each of the perspectives and ERM begins with an understanding of objectives.

For each BSC perspective, measurable KPIs are selected and stretch targets are set.

Through the identification of the risk that is threatening the targets, ERM adds value to the BSC.

Indeed, the organisation can assess the effectiveness of its risk mitigation by monitoring the KPIs.

If a target is not achieved, it indicates that some risks related to the event exist. The same metric can be used for monitoring both strategy and risk (Shenkir, & Walker, 2014).

Nevertheless, organisations need to consider a risk's impact based on not only a departmental dimension (i.e, traditional silo), but also an organisation-wide dimension, which takes into account criteria on process complexity, control effectiveness, and the achievement of an organisation's strategic objectives (e.g., reputation management).

For example, the tragedies of PCR, Texas City refinery, Upper Big Branch mine, Deepwater Horizon, Tazreen Fashions factory and Rana Plaza pointed to a chain of OHS deficiencies but also resulted in significant damage to the reputation of these organisations.

Therefore, a risk of minor OSH implication or low likelihood but with a large impact on the organisation's mission must still be evaluated and escalated to the appropriate decision-makers. Using a standardised process through an ERM allows to easily identify the key health and safety resources within an organisation (Minsky, 2015).

3. OHSMS performance measurements and calculations

OHSMS are based on the continual improvement cycle frequently referred to as the PDCA (Plan-Do-Check-Act) cycle which integrates performance measurement and strategic planning not only to improve management but also set the foundation for implementing results-based OHSMS ('figure 4').

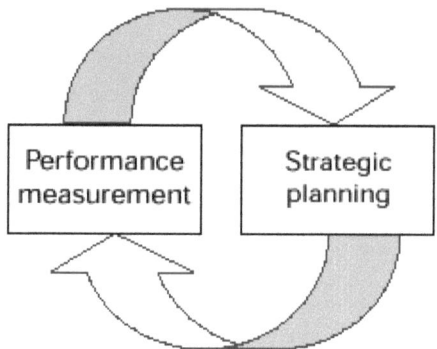

Figure 4: The circle of strategic planning and performance measurement
(Dusenbury, 2000)

A prerequisite of an effective OHSMS is that it should be based on SMART (Specific, Measurable, Attainable, Realistic/Relevant and Time-bound) KPIs. This means that regular checks on progress can be made at appropriate intervals against a defined performance standard (Health and Safety Executive UK, 2001).

Therefore, KPIs are important to measure the efficiency of the OHSMS ('Figure 5') and must be categorised into two types: lagging and leading indicators ('Figure 6').

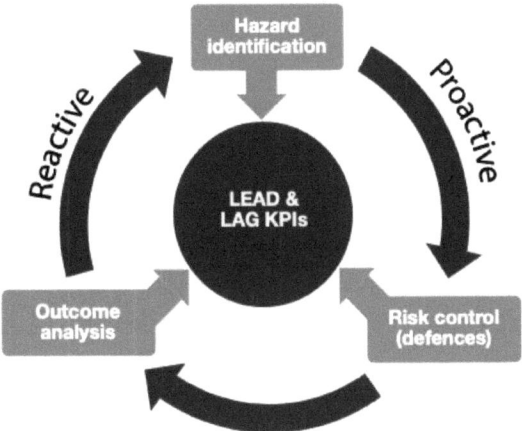

Figure 5: The cycle of OHSMS (Safety Australia, 2017)

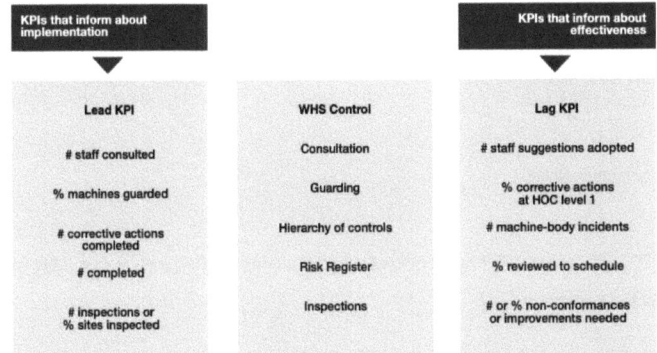

Figure 6: Evaluating the implementation and effectiveness of OHSMS Controls (Safe Work Australia, 2017).

3.1 Lag indicators

Lag KPIs are outcome indicators reflecting generally the results of past actions and are used to report on the effectiveness of OHSMS.

3.1.1 Total Recordable Injury (and illness) (TRI)

TRI focuses on frequency by calculating the sum of fatalities, Lost Time Injuries (LTI), Medical Treated Injuries (MTI) and Restricted Work Injuries (RWI).

Then, TRI frequency rates (TRIFR) are calculated as TRI per one million hours worked ('Figure 7').

3.1.2 Days away / restricted / transfer rate (DART)

$$\frac{\text{Number of all recordable injuries in a 12-month period}}{\text{Total hours worked by all staff in same 12-month period}} \times 1{,}000{,}000 = \text{TRIFR}$$

Figure 7: TRIFR

DART captures a broader range of events and is a comparable measure that TRIs that affect the workplace.

Unlike LTFIR, it is less likely to create dysfunctional consequences such as under-reporting and data manipulation (Safe Work Australia, 2017).

Therefore, DART is the sum of incidents that resulted in:
- one or more days lost (see LTI below), or
- one or more days on restricted work duties, or

- that resulted in an employee being transferred to a different role or duty in the organisation,

per one million hours worked ('figure 8')

Editor's note: Image has been removed due to copyright reasons.

Figure 8: DART Rate (OSHAcademy Safety and Health Training, 2018)

3.1.3 Lost Time Injury (LTI)

LTI frequency rates (LTIFR) 'have, over time, become the cornerstone of mainstream injury reporting and the benchmark against which organisational, industry and national comparisons are made' (O'Neill et al., 2013). Like DART, this KPI focuses on productivity disruption (Work Safe Australia, 2017).

Therefore, LTI represents the sum of work-related fatality, injury or illness outcomes that have resulted in an individual being deemed fully unfit for work for a period of an entire work shift or more, at any time after the day or shift on which the injury or illness occurred, irrespective of whether a workers' compensation claim has been lodged or not (Safe Work Australia, 2017).

Meanwhile, the calculation of LTIFR represents the number of LTIs per one million hours worked (' Figure 9').

| Number of lost time injuries in a 12-month period | / | Total hours worked by all staff in same 12-month period | x | 1,000,000 | = | LTIFR |

Figure 9: LTIFR

Lag KPIs are negative performance indicators (NPI) because they do not measure the success of the OHSMS but its failure.

For example, LTIs provide little indication of the cost or severity of injuries and are often manipulated.

Indeed, it is not unusual that investigations reveal the company had a good record (i.e., low LTIFR) before a particular event that caused a fatality or serious injuries (Hopkins, 1994)

Meanwhile, Australian Occupational Health and Safety Representatives (2015) claim that: 'Such data is unlikely to provide a valid indicator for either the severity or cost of those work health and safety failures that result in lost time... or the success of work health and safety controls and initiatives.

Furthermore, Hopkins (1994) observes that LTIs are more sensitive to claims and injury management processes than to real changes in safety performance;

Only a few injuries may occur in a workplace annually, and variations from year to year are likely to be due to chance, rather than due to any improvement in the levels of safety with no information about how well the most serious safety hazards are being managed.

3.2 Leading indicators

The alternatives to outcome indicators are positive performance indicators (PPI) or OHS inputs (i.e., effort) and their measures reflect the implementation of OHS controls

For example, PPI may include the number of safety audits conducted, the percentage of sub-standard conditions identified and corrected, the percentage of employees with adequate OHS training, peer to peer observation behaviour based safety (BBS), management safety walk (SWA), risk control effectiveness (RCE) or lessons learned.

Therefore, they are the action steps that a workplace can take to prevent future incidents and measuring them is a great predictor of incidents (Occupational Health and Safety Representatives (AU), 2015).

However, the challenge is measuring PPI reliably and consistently across different industries to create a benchmark.

So far, only the Institute of Work and Health in Canada has developed a tool with great potential for application.

Indeed, in ' figure 10' the Organisational Performance Metric (OPM) is an eight-item questionnaire to measure the perceptions of staff regarding the value of, and emphasis is given, to their organisation's OHSMS with the results being benchmarked against similar industries or multi-sectors

Editor's note: Image has been removed due to copyright reasons.

Figure 10: OPM (Institute for Work & Health, 2016).

4. Conclusion

PPI allows the OHSMS performance to be measured by outcome indicators.

Therefore, the OHSMS performance should not rely on one-dimensional data (e.g., LTIFR) but on multidimensional internal and external data.

Together, lead and lag OHS KPIs inform decisions, from operating choices for frontline managers through to the allocation of resources and analyses of performance at the executive levels of the organisation.

Moreover, the OHSMS should be an integral part of the strategic plan of the organisation and operational risks be scrutinised at the same level of importance than other risks (e.g., financial risks).

References

Balanced Scorecard Institute. (2021, January 22). *Strategic planning basics.* https://
balancedscorecard.org/strategic-planning-basics/

Cooper, E. (n.d.). *The road to ERM: using the Balanced Scorecard to implement
Enterprise Risk Management.* Strategy Management Group. https://
strategymanage.com/wp-content/uploads/pdfs/
UsingBSCforEnterpriseRiskManagemen.pdf

Deloitte. (2017). *Integrating Enterprise Risk Management (ERM) with strategic
planning.* https://www2.deloitte.com/content/dam/Deloitte/us/Documents/
public-sector/us-fed-integrating-erm-with-strategic-planning.pdf

Dusenbury, P. (2000, August 1). *Strategic planning and performance measurement.*
https://webarchive.urban.org/publications/310259.html

Health and Safety Executive UK. (2001, December). *A guide to measuring health &
safety performance.* HSE: Information about health and safety at work. https://
www.hse.gov.uk/opsunit/perfmeas.pdf

Hopkins, A. (1994). *The limits of lost time injury frequency rates.* Work Safe Australia.
https://www.safeworkaustralia.gov.au/system/files/documents/1702/
positiveperformanceindicators_ohs_beyondlosttimeinjuriespart_1-
issues_1994_archivepdf.pdf

Institute for Work & Health. (2016, January). *IWH Organizational Performance Metric.*
https://www.iwh.on.ca/sites/iwh/files/iwh/tools/iwh-opm_questionnaire_2016-
v2.pdf

International Organization for Standardization. (2018). *ISO 31000:2018 Risk management — Guidelines*. ISO - International Organization for Standardization. https://www.iso.org/obp/ui/#iso:std:iso:31000:ed-2:v1:en

Meng, X., & Yahanpath, N. (n.d.). *The value ambiguity of ERM: The case study of Pike River Coal Mine*. https://cdn.auckland.ac.nz/assets/business/about/our-departments/od-accounting-finance/NZMAS%20Symposium%202016/The%20value%20ambiguity%20of%20ERM_Noel%20Yahanpath.pdf

Minsky, S. (2015, January 26). *Assessing Reputational risk for occupational safety & health*. ERM Software. https://www.logicmanager.com/resources/erm/assessing-reputational-risk-occupational-safety-health/

Occupational Health and Safety Representatives (AU). (2015). *Measure health and safety performance*. OHS Reps. https://www.ohsrep.org.au/measure_health_and_safety_performance

OSHAcademy Safety and Health Training. (2018). *Calculating OSHA DART and TCIR rates - Free online training*. Free Access | Online Safety Training | OSHA Training | OSHAcademy. https://www.oshatrain.org/courses/mods/708m6.html#

O'Neill, S., Martinov-Bennie, N., & Cheung, A. (2013, November). *Issues in the measurement and reporting of work health and safety performance: a review*. Work Safe Australia. https://www.safeworkaustralia.gov.au/system/files/documents/1703/issues-measurement-reporting-whs-performance.pdf

Royal Commission into the Pike River Mine Tragedy. (2012, October 30). *Royal Commission Report*. Royal Commission into the Pike River Mine Tragedy - pikeriver.royalcommission.govt.nz. https://pikeriver.royalcommission.govt.nz

Safe Work Australia. (2017, March). *Measuring and reporting on work health and safety*. https://www.safeworkaustralia.gov.au/system/files/documents/1802/measuring-and-reporting-on-work-health-and-safety.pdf

Shenkir, W. G., & Walker, P. L. (2014). *ERM: Frameworks, elements, and integration | IMA - The association of accountants and financial professionals working in business*. https://www.imanet.org/insights-and-trends/risk-management/enterprise-risk-management?ssopc=1

Stanton, T. H. (2020, September 14). *Overview of ERM*. Thomas H. Stanton – Public Sector Author, Professor, Lawyer. https://thomas-stanton.com/wp-content/uploads/2021/01/Overview-of-ERM-09-14-2020-meeting.pdf

Visual Paradigm. (n.d.). *Using strategy map with balanced scoreboard*. Visual Paradigm Online - Suite of Powerful Tools. https://online.visual-paradigm.com/knowledge/strategic-map/strategy-map-with-balanced-scoreboard/

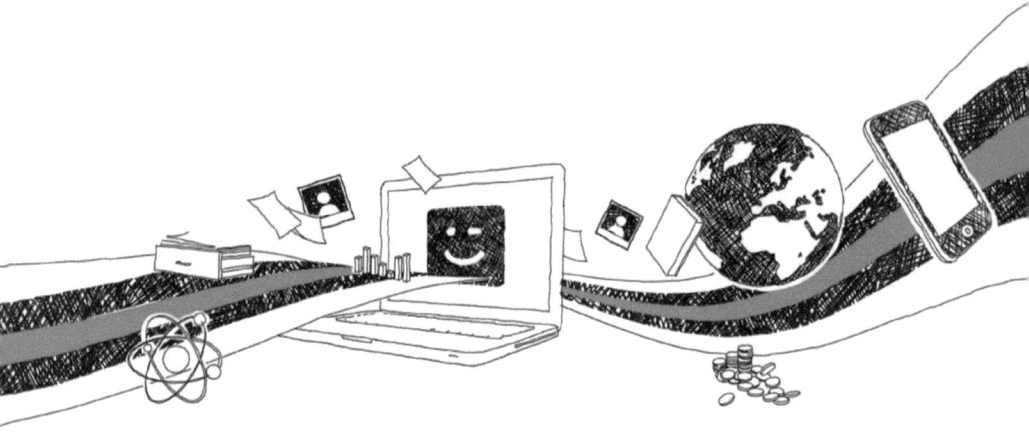
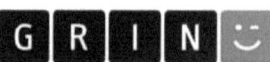